Trigger Point Therapy

Stop Muscle & Joint Pain Naturally with Easy to use Trigger Point Therapy

Volume Two

By

Dermot Farrell

Copyright © 2018 and beyond Dermot Farrell

All Rights Reserved. No part of this publication may be reproduced in any form or by any means, including scanning, photocopying, or otherwise without prior written permission of the copyright holder.

Disclaimer and Terms of Use: The Author and Publisher has strived to be as accurate and complete as possible in the creation of this book, notwithstanding the fact that he does not warrant or represent at any time that the contents within are accurate due to the rapidly changing nature of the Internet. While all attempts have been made to verify information provided in this publication, the Author and Publisher assumes no responsibility for errors, omissions, or contrary interpretation of the subject matter herein. Any perceived slights of specific persons, peoples, or organizations are unintentional. In practical advice books, like anything else in life, there are no guarantees of income made. This book is not intended for use as a source of legal, business, accounting or financial advice. All readers are advised to seek services of competent professionals in legal, business, accounting, and finance field.

First Printing, 2018

MEDICAL DISCLAIMER

The information in this book is not intended to replace professional medical supervision. The information in this book is highly effective and it will definitely reduce the chronic pain issues of nearly every person. In some cases a cure may take place; however, there is no guarantee that physical ailments will be completely cured. Prior to reducing or stopping allopathic medications, do consult with a qualified physician.

Contents

INTRODUCTION TO VOLUME TWO   7

PART ONE – THEORY

CHAPTER ONE - A GUIDE TO SELF TREATMENT   10

HANDS   12

TOOLS   14

PART TWO – PRACTICAL

CHAPTER TWO – NECK AND HEAD PAIN

1. SPLENIUS CAPITAS   17
2. TEMPORALIS   19

CHAPTER THREE – CHEST AND BACK AND SHOULDERS

3.	STERNALIS	22
4.	PECTORALIS MAJOR (STERNAL DIVISION)	23
5.	PECTORALIS MAJOR (CLAVICULAR DIVISION)	24
6.	MULTIFIDUS SPINAE	25
7.	LONGISSIMUS DORSI	27
8.	POSTERIOR CERVICAL	29
9.	INFRASPINATUS	30
10.	DELTOID.	31

CHAPTER FOUR – GLUTES AND LEGS

11. GLUTEUS MINIMUS	34
12. ADDUCTOR LONGUS	36
13. VASTUS MEDIALIS	38
14. TIBIALIS ANTICUS	39
15 BICEPS FEMORIS	42

CHAPTER FIVE – ARMS & HANDS

16. SUPINATOR — 43

17. EXTENSOR CARPIL RADIALIS — 45

18. MIDDLE FINGER EXTENSOR — 47

19. FIRST INTEROSSEOUS — 48

20. ABDUCTOR POLLICIS — 49

Introduction to Volume Two

Following on from the continued success of Trigger Point Therapy Volume One, I decided to write a follow-up volume, in order to provide even more useful trigger points for your use. And just like volume one, this book is free of fluff and is written in a very straightforward way with easy to follow instructions and helpful pictures and diagrams. Also the trigger points have been labelled under body parts in order to make it most helpful for you.

The term trigger point sounds somewhat exotic, so what exactly are trigger points and how can they help you improve your health?

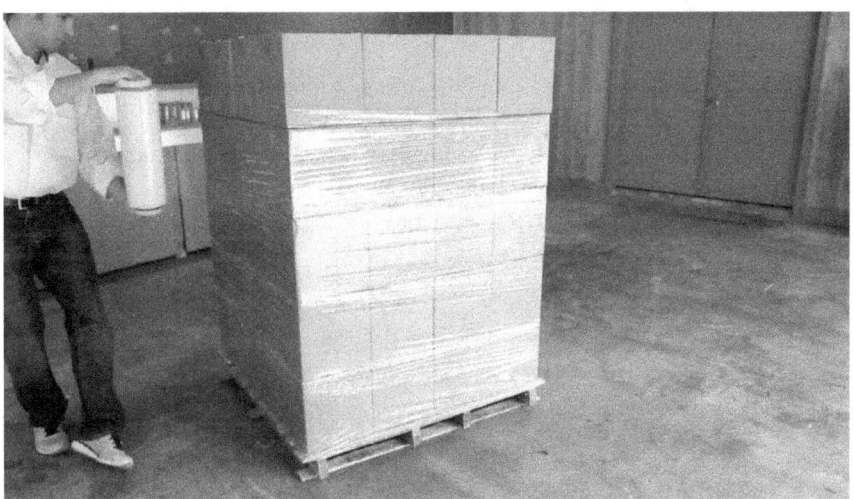

The whole idea of trigger points is that pain is distributed along the fascia tissue, which runs over the muscles, ligaments, and tendons like a web. We tend to think of fascia as been the upholstery in your car, but also fascia is a technical term used to refer to tissue which encapsulates the muscles, ligaments, and tendons.

On a simple level the fascia keeps the tissues of the body in place, otherwise, if say you were cut, everything would just fall out! Maybe a nice way to think about the fascia is to visualize it as if it were that plastic wrap which freight forwarders wrap around pallets, in order to keep everything in place.

So this is the primary role of fascia, but fascia also has a secondary role, whereby if a person has pain in one part of the body, caused by either an injury of some sort, or an imbalance, the body processes the pain by inflaming the muscles, ligaments and tendons, which in turn press against the fascia and often result in a pain in the fascia quite a distance away from the epicentre of the pain.

So where trigger points come into play is that that ache that you might have in your leg or hip or lower back etc., you know the one which just won't go away; well if you trigger point it, often you will get near instantaneous relief and the reason for this is because the trigger points relieve tension, not only in this area of the body but also back along the fascia itself to the origin point of the physical disturbance.

Trigger points can work almost as if by magic, but really there is nothing miraculous about them, rather they are simply highly effective pressure points which release pain and imbalances from the body!

In this book volume two I have left out the theory chapters, if you want more theory then refer back to volume one, but I have left in the chapter entitled " A Guide to Self Treatment", as even if you have not read volume one you can still work the magic of trigger points by yourself, by following this instructional chapter and then picking out trigger points which are relevant to the pain area which you are looking to work upon.

Part One – Theory

Chapter One - A Guide to Self Treatment

Trigger points are generally used by professional therapists, however, they can also be used by individuals in order to release tension in the trigger points.

While there are obvious restrictions, regarding what we can self-release (after all a trained professional, applying force from a strategic angle, is going to have more success at getting into hard to reach areas), a lot of physical tensions.

The thing to bear in mind, however, is that trigger points will not release if we use a namby-pamby approach. If you have ever been to a physical therapist, then you will remember the pain, yes pain is the appropriate word here. The degree of relief felt is largely proportional to three factors:

1. The willingness of the patient to undergo discomfort (even pain)
2. Knowledge of the practitioner
3. The frequency of the treatment

Just think about these three factors, for a minute. If we are willing to undergo discomfort, then a greater level of release will be felt. But to undergo a horrendous session of Self Myofascial Release (SMR), whereby a great relief is felt and then only to leave everything alone for weeks until the problem becomes chronic again, is a complete waste of time. Also, the opposite of this is a namby-pamby approach, whereby we go through the motions, but we never really get the release, in the first place, is also a complete waste of our time and effort.

So, the approach, which we need to take, is one whereby we are willing to push enough to provide a release (but not necessarily a mind-blowing hour and a half long, sweating, agonising one), but equally importantly we should carry out daily sessions. Maybe not daily sessions, of the one body part, maybe split the body parts over several sessions, but the idea is to do ten to twenty minutes a day regularly. When we take this approach, little by little, we get the relief which we need, as the physical imbalances slowly right themselves.

Another factor, which must also be remembered, is that physical massage is not enough. These physical imbalances usually arose out of lifestyle imbalances, over a long period of time, and lifestyle changes also need to be made. For example, say you have a soleus problem with your calf, and have all sorts of aches and pains; sure the trigger points will aid relief, but maybe you have to change your shoes, get corrective sole supports for your fallen arches and change some aspects of your walking gait, maybe you will even have to change how you sit and do some other exercises, such as Pilates or yoga, for example, and maybe some core exercises, so as to rebalance your posture, only then will a complete healing take place.

So we have to think in terms of ten to twenty minutes a day, over a period of months practicing these SMR strategies, while also working on our various imbalances and lifestyle changes. This might sound extreme, as we are living in the age of "take a pill and forget about it", but seriously if you want to get permanent relief from orthopedic stiffness and pain, the approach to take is one of working through imbalances, over time. Take this approach and great results will take place!

Finally, looking at release again, we have to be willing to grab and squeeze the muscle and fascia.

Hands

We can use our forefinger, thumb, forefinger and thumb or hand grab.

Forefinger: We can use our forefinger to poke around. This is great from a diagnostic point of view, as the easiest way to find a trigger point is to poke around until pain is felt, but it's usually lacking the necessary power to bring about release.

Thumb: Our thumbs are really strong, so obviously they are good at prodding into hard to reach places, and gaining relief.

Forefinger and Thumb: This is a great combination, whereby we can grasp the area and apply pressure to the trigger point, for fast effective relief.

Knuckles: Knuckles are a really great way of getting a deep, sharp, localised effect into a specific area.

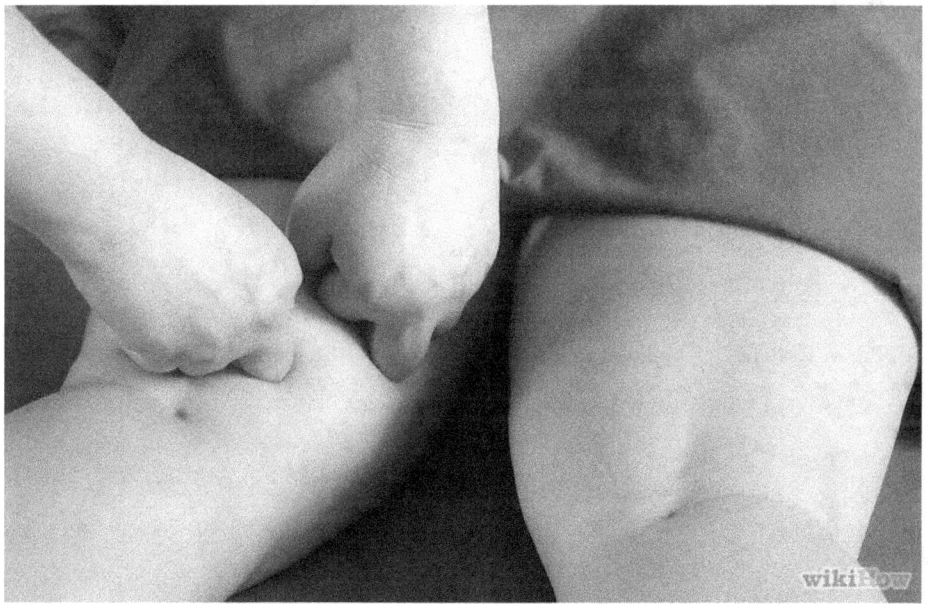

Picture courtesy of wikihow

Hand Grab: This can be a useful technique, whereby we can gain even more leverage. A really good example of hand grab can be applied on our upper traps, whereby we aim for the midmost point and grab the trap as if were about to lift up a six pack, but instead we grab, hold and squeeze.

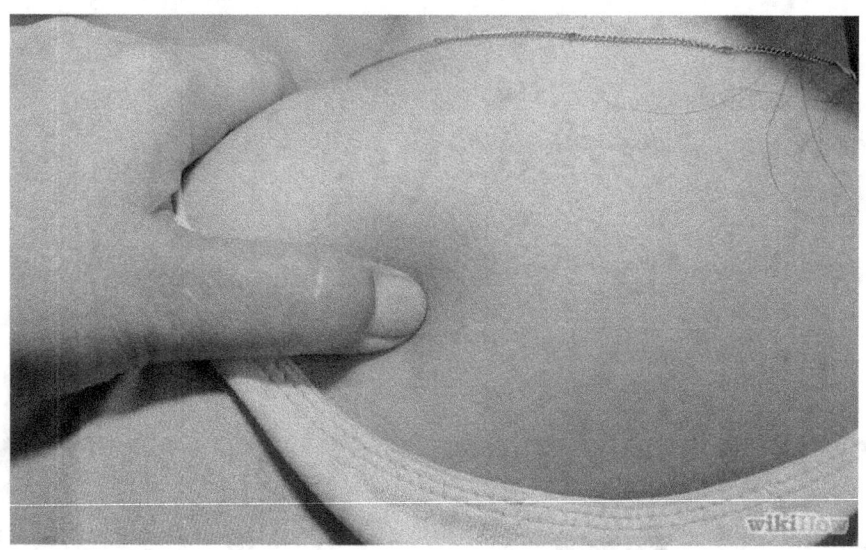

Picture courtesy of wikihow

Tools

Foam Roller: The foam roller is probably the most famous SMR tool, and simply it is a roller with foam on it!

How do we use it effectively?

Simply find the trigger point and roll back and forth over it until release comes. This is ideal for big areas, such as legs, lower back, upper back, hip area etc. The key is to keep rolling and working towards getting a tighter squeeze in this area. Once you get into it, a noticeable feeling of ache and pressure will build up and simply follow the ache as it slowly releases. Work at it for ten to fifteen minutes, from a variety of angles and then let it go until tomorrow, remember Rome was not built in a day!

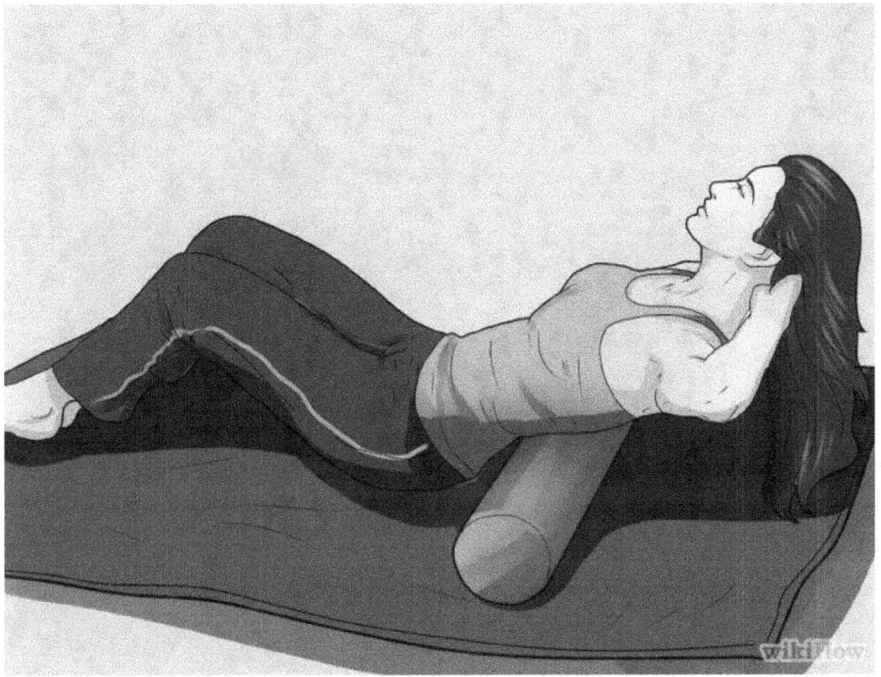

Picture courtesy of wikihow

Massage ball: The massage ball (it doesn't have to be a massage ball, as any type of hardball, rubber ball etc., will do the job), is ideal for those hard to reach places, such as shoulders, chest, and very specific parts of the back, Think of the foam roller as something large and dull in operation, whereas the ball is small and sharp, so it's a better tool for getting into hard to reach places, where the pain is more localised. In many ways, its operation is similar to knuckle massage, but obviously, it allows us to access parts of our own body, which we could not access via our knuckles.

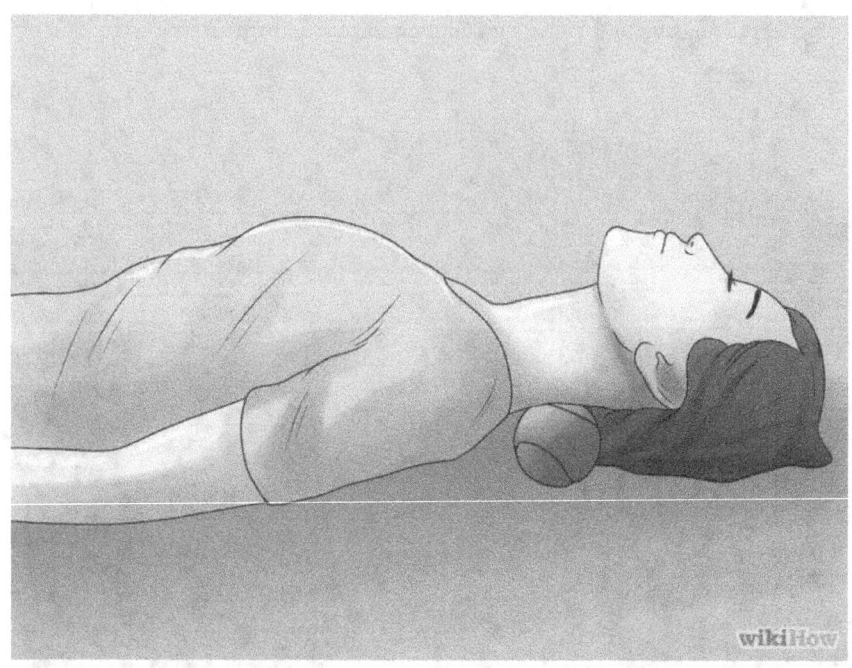

Picture courtesy of wikihow

Part Two – Practical

Chapter Two – Neck and Head Pain

1. *Splenius capitas*

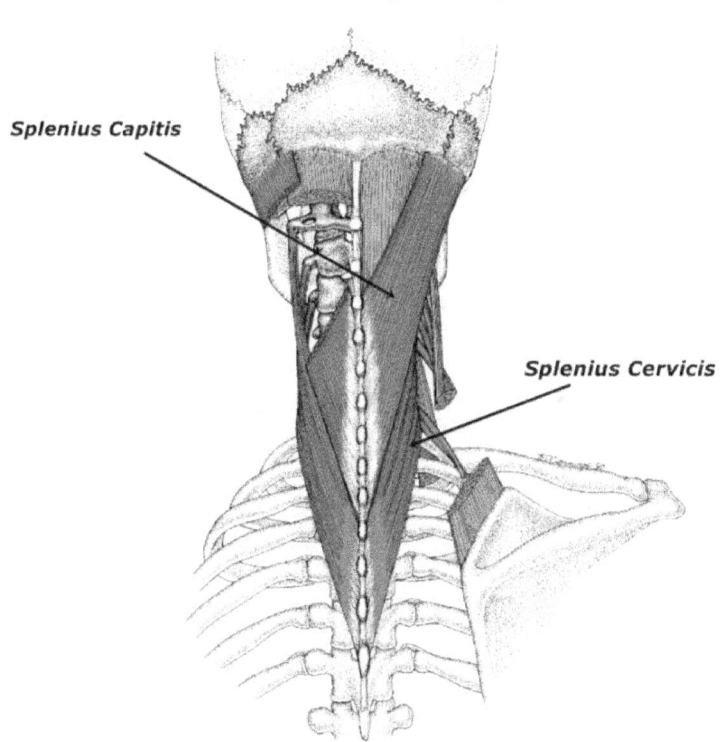

Description:
The splemius capitas is a muscle which runs from the upper back and cervical area of the neck upto the top of the head. The fibers run upwards and outwards

and inserts under the sternomastoid muscle, into the mastoid process behind the ear and at the base of the skull.

Function:

The function of this muscle is to stabilize the neck, as there are two muscles each one running along the side of the neck. These muscles stabilize the neck and help to move the help the head to move backwards.

Symptoms:

Splenius capitas problems result in pain and throbbing sensations in the top of the head. Often sensations of burning or tinkling are also found in the upper head region.

Trigger Point Therapy:

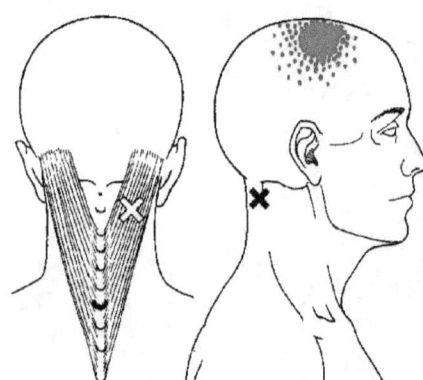

To release this point, simply direct pressure onto the relevant point as seen in the diagram below.

A second way to work the point is to stretch it while moving the head forward and away from the side being treated. You can also use a rub or muscle pain spry on the neck area before trying the stretch. Importantly you should be able to move your neck forward, back and sideways without restriction.

If you feel a restriction in your neck accompanied by a throbbing pain it might be that this point needs to be released. It's certainly worth trying to release the point and then see how you get on.

Start out by using pressure on the point first and if some release is felt then try stretching the neck out gently. Releasing a point with pressure will also require a firm press but when stretching the neck try not to put undue pressure on the neck as this could make it worse.

2. Temporalis

Description:
The temporalis is a fan-shaped muscle situated on the side of the head. It originates on the temporal bone of the skull and its fibers converge on the jawbone. In simple English the temporalis muscle runs from the side of the head down to the jawbone, just take a look at the diagram below. The temporalis trigger point is found just above the temple bone, a bone which runs from the upper ear to the eye socket. As the diagram reveals there are four sub-points which all lie along the length of the temporalis muscles and which can be stimulated.

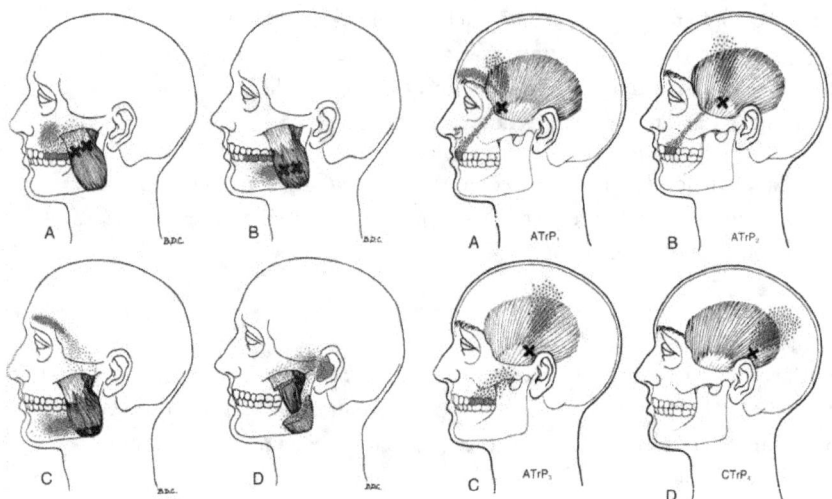

Function:

The main function of the temporalis muscle is to close the mouth. Its upper fiber can be felt above the temple when the jaw is clenched.

Symptoms:

Various complaints can be found in this muscle. Uneven teeth and injuries to the face commonly have an effect here. Also **Trigeminal neuralgia** (a condition whereby one side of the face suffers from disturbing nerve pain), can also cause problems here. Stress and tension can also have an effect on the face. So symptoms can vary from pain to weird sensations to a general disturbance within the facial area.

Trigger Point Therapy:

The easiest way to get going with this point is to press your forefinger against your cheekbone and then pull your finger back towards your ear. Depending upon the size of your head, approximately half to one inch away from your ear simply slide your forefinger up over the cheekbone and then you will feel the soft fleshy are which is known as the temple.

Now as the diagram shows there are actually four trigger points running along this muscle, from near the eye and then right back to an area just past your ear. The approach which has mentioned above is a good starting point. You can then search along this line which runs just over the cheekbone and search out for sensitive areas and wherever you feel a sensitive spot, simply press and hold for about twenty seconds or so. Release and repeat for twenty seconds and do so several times before moving onto the other sub-points.

Chapter Three – Chest and Back and Shoulders

3. Sternalis

Description:

The sternalis is an area of tissue which covers the sternum (breastplate)

Function:

It has no apparent function other than it's a general piece of fascia and like all fascia, it helps to hold muscles ligaments and tendons in place.

Symptoms:

This is a good point for pain in the chest area and particular any kind of chest bone pain.

Trigger Point Therapy:

This point is more or less an intuitive point. Simply trace a line from the beginning of the sternum up several inches until you find the most sensitive part of the sternum and then simply press for twenty seconds and release, take a few seconds out and then repeat several times.

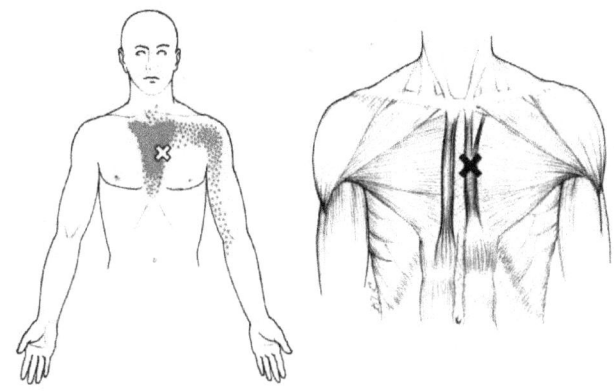

4. Pectoralis major (Sternal Division)

Description:

This is the large triangular part of the pectoralis muscle (breast muscle), which runs from the ribcage up to the shoulder joint at the edge of the upper arm.

Function:

This part of the pectoralis muscle's function is to lift the arm forward and across the midline of the body. It also helps to rotate the arm inwards.

Symptoms:

Pain in the chest muscle, in particular towards the outer arm and feelings of tension. This can arise from working out such as lifting weights or doing push-ups, but also tension and pain here can originate as a consequence of blunt trauma to the body, such as minor or major accidents.

Trigger Point Therapy:

To locate this point, take a look at the diagram below and then try to grab your pectoralis muscle as if you were trying to pinch something. The thumb should be on the pectoralis muscle, while the forefinger and middle fingers should in the region of the armpit. Have a feel around until you find some tenderness and then work at pressing for twenty seconds and then let go for ten seconds and then repeat several times on this same point. You can also have a feel around for what are named in Traditional Chinese Medicine as "Local Points", a local point been anywhere where pain and tension is held in the muscles and fascia.

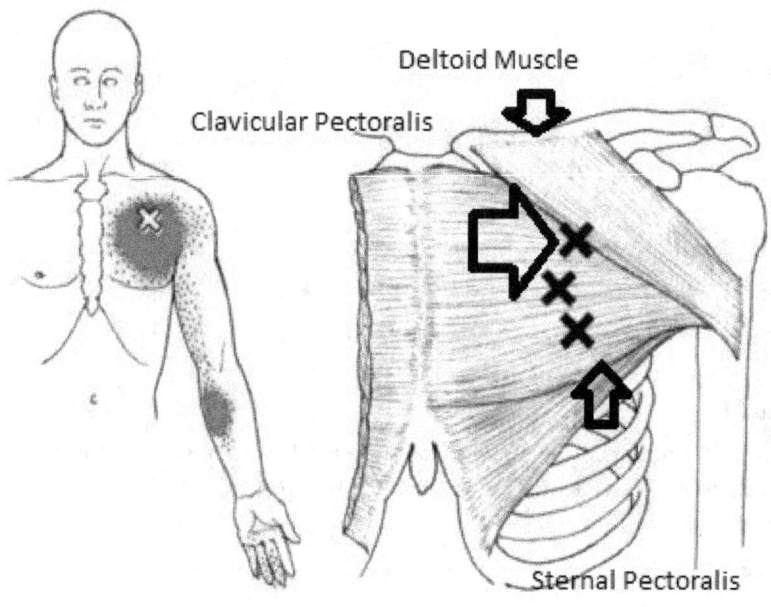

5. *Pectoralis major (Clavicular Division)*

Description:

This part of the pectoralis muscle runs from the inner half of the collarbone down to the upper part of the shoulder insertion. This trigger point of the pectoralis is basically slightly higher up than sternal section of the pectoralis muscle.

Function:

This muscle helps with bending and raising the upper arm.

Symptoms:

Pain in the breast area radiating out towards the arm and often relates to mental-emotional stress.

Trigger Point Therapy:

The way to differentiate between sternal and clavicular pectoralis muscles is to raise your arm and then get someone to stop you raising your arm above shoulder level. When you do so, you shall note that the clavicular section of the pectoralis muscle activates. Whereas the sternal part of the pectoralis muscle activates much lower, as we try and hold our arm out near nipple level.

Where then do we press for trigger point relief?

Well have a feel around near the very upper part of your pectoralis muscle near the shoulder/upper arm, near the area were the deltoid passes over the pectoralis muscle, just take a look at the picture again.

6. *Multifidus spinae*

Description:

The multifidis spinae are a series of strips of muscles which run parallel to the spine from the base of the spine right up to the neck.

Function:

These are postural muscles which control core stability of the spinal joints. They also have an effect on side bending and rotating torso movements.

Symptoms:

Pain in this region. The pain could be anywhere, so rather than getting hung up on a particular point think in terms of potential "local points", points which can shift slightly from person to person.

Trigger Point Therapy:

The easiest way to get the points here is to grab either your waist if the pain is in this area and then squeeze with your thumb from behind and your fingers from the front of your torso. If the pain is not located near the waist area then ask a helper to feel around the back area near the spine and whenever you feel pain or tension, get them to squeeze and release this point. Also, stretching can also be good idea here when combined with trigger points.

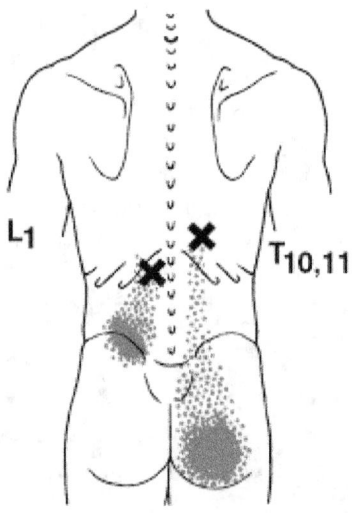

7. *Longissimus dorsi*

Description:

The longissimus dorsi belong to the erector spinae muscles (the muscles which lie along the lower end of the back muscles which help to bend over or stand back up while keeping one's legs straight.)

Function:

These muscles help the spine to bend forward, back or sideways.

Symptoms:

Pain anywhere from the eight-rib down to the buttock. The nature of fascia been what it is, the pain can just as easily be nebulous as it can be specific.

Trigger Point Therapy:

Feel your lower back near your spine and press the area of pain or sensitivity. Foam rolling can be good and also a very good approach is to take either a massage ball (baseball, cricket ball or hard rubber ball will work easily well). When using a massage ball, place the ball against the wall and press your back against the ball and squeeze hard, release and repeat several times.

Also, do not get hung up on one point, rather feel a sensitive spot and work on it a few times, then move around your back. Often you will find that as the pain releases, that the pain starts moving around either the lower, mid back or the buttocks. So feel your way through the tension and work towards a release.

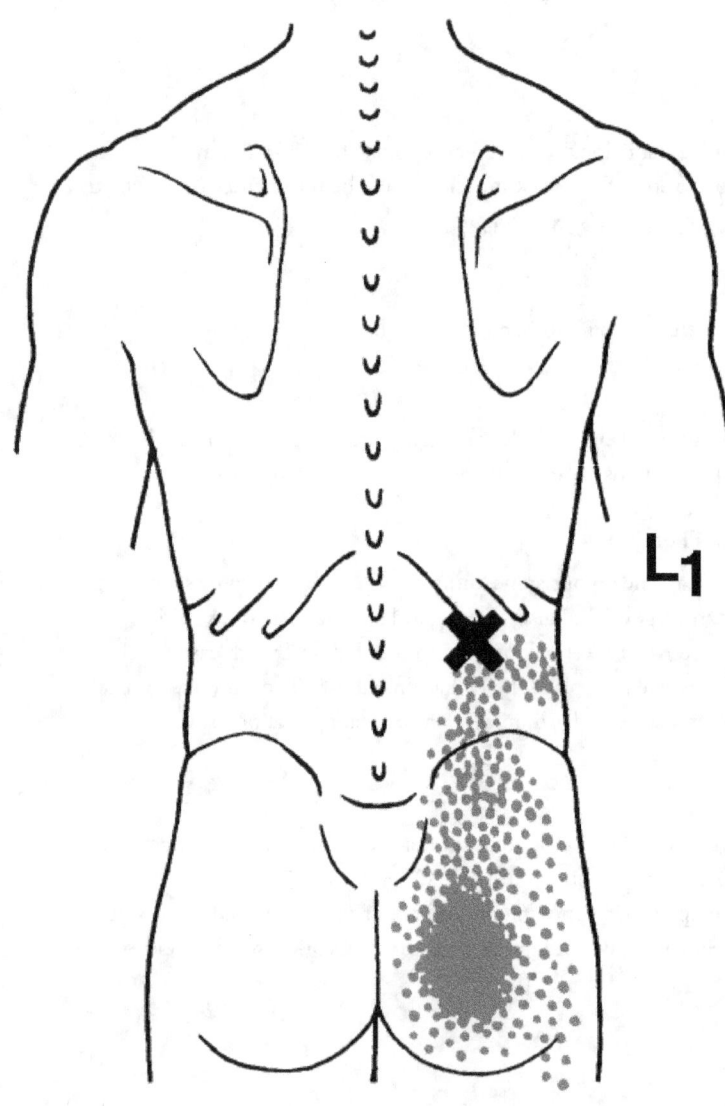

8. Posterior cervical

Description:

These muscles attach from the lower cervical and upper thoracic region.

Function:

The purpose of these muscles is to help move the head forwards back and sideways.

Symptoms:

Pain in the neck, base of the skull or inability to move the neck fully.

Trigger Point Therapy:

The posterior cervical muscles tend to overlap each other, so a certain variety of movements will be required to get a good trigger release. Probably fingers and thumb are the best way to go and often a fair amount of pressure will be required, usually applied towards the back of the neck near the base of the skull. As always squeeze for twenty to thirty seconds and release, take a few seconds of and release and work away through the areas of tension and tenderness.

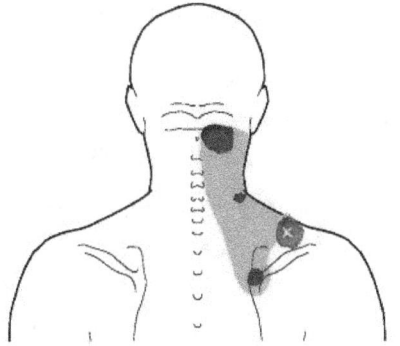
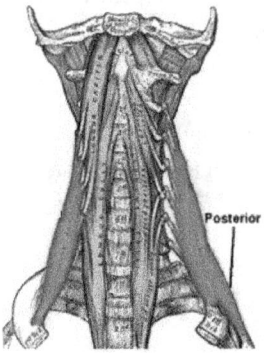

9. Infraspinatus

Description:

This is a thick triangular muscle arising out of the inner border and the posterior surface of the shoulder blade. It runs towards and inserts into the rear part of the upper arm.

Function:

It is one of several muscles which help to stabilize the upper arm into the shoulder joint.

Symptoms:

Pain in the outer and upper arm and often a sensation of having a frozen shoulder can occur.

Trigger Point Therapy:

The trigger point(s) here are found on the shoulder blade and the easiest way to reach there, if you are working on yourself, then reach around with the other hand and grab the head of your shoulder while trying to squeeze the back part of your shoulder blade.

Now there is no exact trigger point, rather you have to feel around and look for areas of tension. If you can get a helper to help you with this, then all the better. The use of a massage ball or any other hardball is once again useful here, whereby you place the ball between the back of your shoulder blade and a wall and simply press back against the wall, hold for a few seconds, release and repeat and then move back and forth and up and down around the area of the shoulder blade until a good degree of release is achieved.

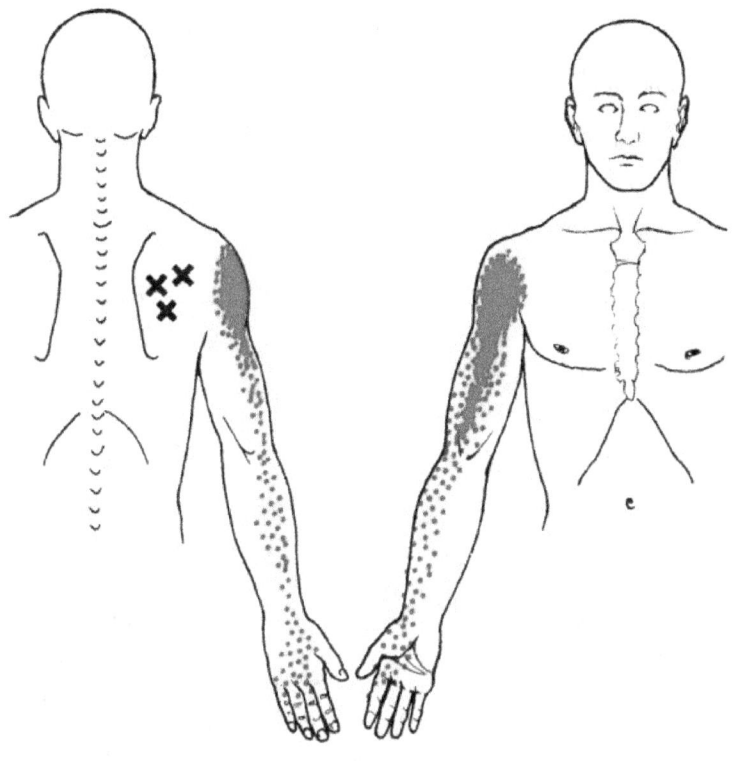

10. Deltoid.

Description:

The deltoid muscles are three muscles which connect the shoulder to the body and the upper arm. They can be split into anterior, medial and posterior (front, middle and rear).

Function:

Each one works at achieving a range of motion in that particular arc of movement, either rising the arm up, moving it out to the side or pulling it back in a rowing movement.

Symptoms:

Atypically shoulder pain stiffens and frozen shoulder usually is in just one plane of motion.

Trigger Point Therapy:

There are actually several points, so just look at the diagram below.

The front trigger point is found by lifting your arm upwards and outwards in a medial (sideways) direction, while at the same time feeling the area between the front and middle deltoid muscle. When the arm reaches around shoulder height, or just over shoulder height you should be able with the finger of your other hand, to feel the line between each deltoid muscle. Then feel around and look out for an area of sensitivity and once you find it then work it with your forefinger.

There are also two points on the medial delt, which can be found by either working around the raised arm all over the middle delt muscle or getting someone to do this manipulation for you.

You don't have to keep your arm raised, this is simply to help location.

Of course you might find that raising your arm is impossible, in which case simply feel around the front and middle deltoid muscles until you can feel an area of extreme tenderness and then work to release the tension.

Once again local points (points which are not official points, rather they are points unique to you were tension in the fascia has built up) are useful here.

Other tricks include using a muscle cream with some eucalyptus in it to help move the arm and of course, for extreme cases, you can begin by taken an ibuprofen twenty minutes beforehand and then rubbing in a muscle cream before beginning the sessions. The reason for this is to relax the muscle and then work at getting the muscle's to move.

The key to healing muscles, in general, is to trigger release in the fascia and then promote movement. And this is particularly so in the deltoids, where frozen shoulder can be very debilitating.

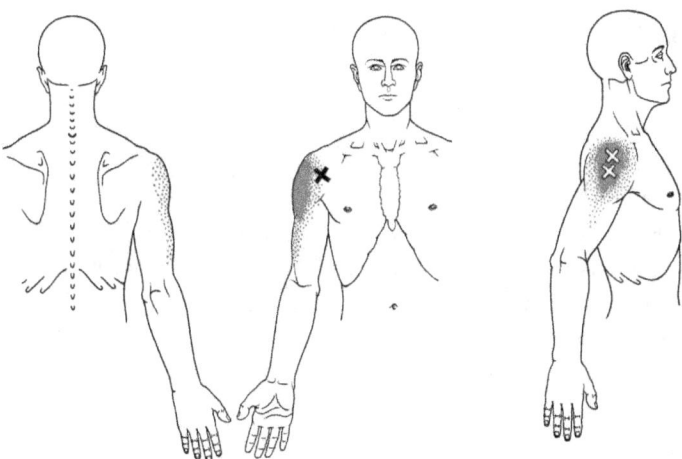

Chapter Four – Glutes and Legs

11. Gluteus Minimus

Description:

There are three glutei muscles (muscles of the bottom) and this one is the smallest. It runs alongside the pelvis and it originates from the upper outer rim of the pelvis and runs downwards to insert into the front outer upper surface of the leg.

Function:

This muscle raises the legs and aids internal rotation of the leg.

Symptoms:

While a small muscle the gluteus minimus can cause a lot of problems and is often difficult to identify.

It results in pain in the lower back, bottom rear thigh and calf. Also it can mimic sciatica pain. And can often result in pain radiating out to other trigger points such as, hamstrings, quadriceps, tensor fascia latae, peroneal and gastrocnemius muscle groups.

Trigger Point Therapy:

There are several trigger points in this area, the main ones been posterior gluteus minimus trigger, which is in the rear part of the muscle, and the lateral gluteus minimus trigger, which lies between the outer rim of the pelvic bone and the hip joint, about two thirds of the way up.

The two lateral points can be found in the anterior fibers (side of the bottom) and are vertically aligned a few inches above the hip joint. So the easiest way to treat this area is to grab your hip between your thumb, middle and forefingers and then squeeze until you can feel the trigger point activate, you can also use a massage ball or foam roller if you like.

As for the posterior trigger points, they lie in the posterior fibers which lie in a radial pattern which follows the hip crest arc, but which are found about several inches below it. In order to locate these points, try and grab your glute (bottom muscle) and feel around near the hip joint until you find an area of tenderness.

Tension in the glutes if often hidden and will require a fairly rigorous approach to both find and then release the tension. Do not be afraid to really put pressure on these points, as although a little painful it will bring about a lot of relief to leg, bottom and lower back symptoms.

Also lower back pain can often follow due to an imbalance of the glutes (the glutes are not firing, therefore, they are not carrying the load) which overloads the back, so if you are having back issues and pain in the glute area, make a point of working on lower back trigger points as well as glute points.

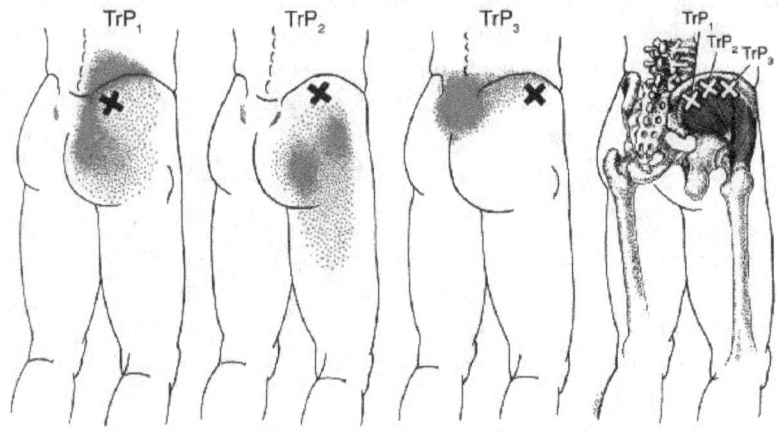

12. Adductor longus

Description:

This is a triangular muscle which extends from the pubic bone and runs downwards and outwards to insert into the middle third of the inner side of the thigh bone.

Function:

This muscle helps to lift the upper leg and is required for abduction of the leg (bringing the leg inwards and across the midline of the body)

Symptoms:

There are two trigger points here with the first one causing pain in the muscle itself and the second one resulting in pain in the front of the hip joint, down the inside if the thigh just above the knee. This pain can be irritating and can often mimic hip pain.

Trigger Point Therapy:

Star by finding the end of the pelvic bone in the crotch area and then move your hand forward a few inches onto your thigh, you should feel a sensitive area this is the second trigger point and the first trigger point is about two inches higher, so simply lift your hand up by around two inches and you will find the first trigger point.

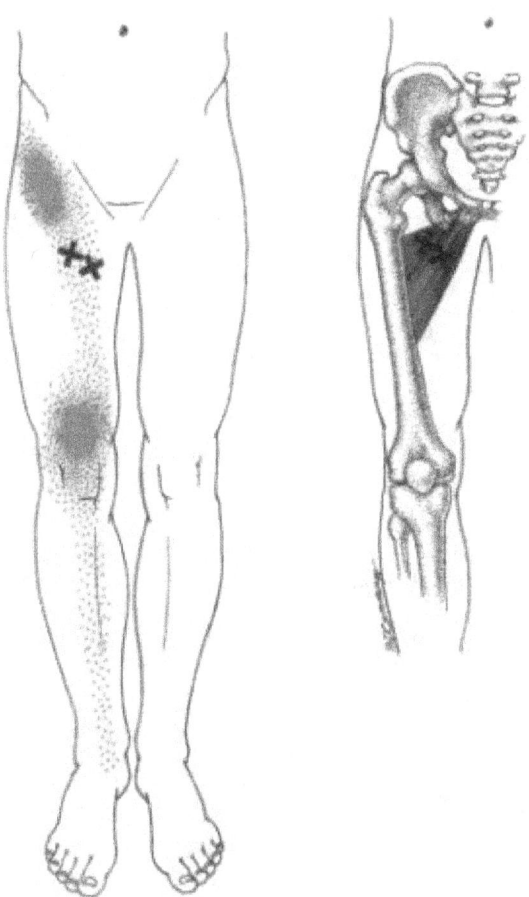

13. Vastus medialis

Description:

This muscle lies on the inner side of the thigh. It originates near the pelvis and extends to just past the kneecap, where this muscle bulges in the case of people who do a lot of leg exercises, this muscle is also known as the knee flexor.

Function:

It helps to straighten the knee and stabilize the joint. If you ever use a leg extension machine then this is the main muscle at work.

Symptoms:

Pain in the kneecap and often pain which feels as if it is radiating out of the knee, also a pain in the inner thigh.

Trigger Point Therapy:

The trigger point here is just above the bony upper part of the knee. Just prior to the kneecap itself is a bony outcrop, just prior to this is the trigger point. It is very easy to work this point via thumb pressure.

There is also a second trigger point about half way up the muscle which can be found by probing with the thumb around the mid part of the inner thigh.

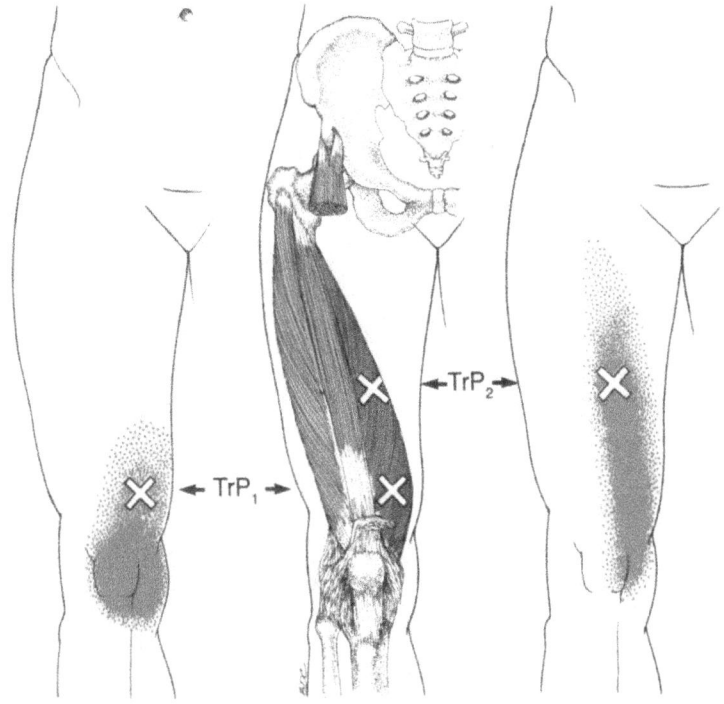

14. Tibialis anticus

Description:

This is the muscle which runs down the front outer part of our calf before crossing over and ending up connecting with the big toe.

Function:

It pulls the foot up towards the knee and also it helps the big toe to rotate. This trigger point is also acupuncture point stomach 36. You can find it by finding the edge of the kneecap and then going down four fingers in width down and here is the point about half an inch from the shin bone. So take one hand and place it

39

horizontally under your knee cap and just under it about half an inch from the shin bone is st 36.

Symptoms:

Pain in the shins, shin splints and pain down into the big toe.

Trigger Point Therapy:

Simple press hard with either your thumb or forefinger for release.

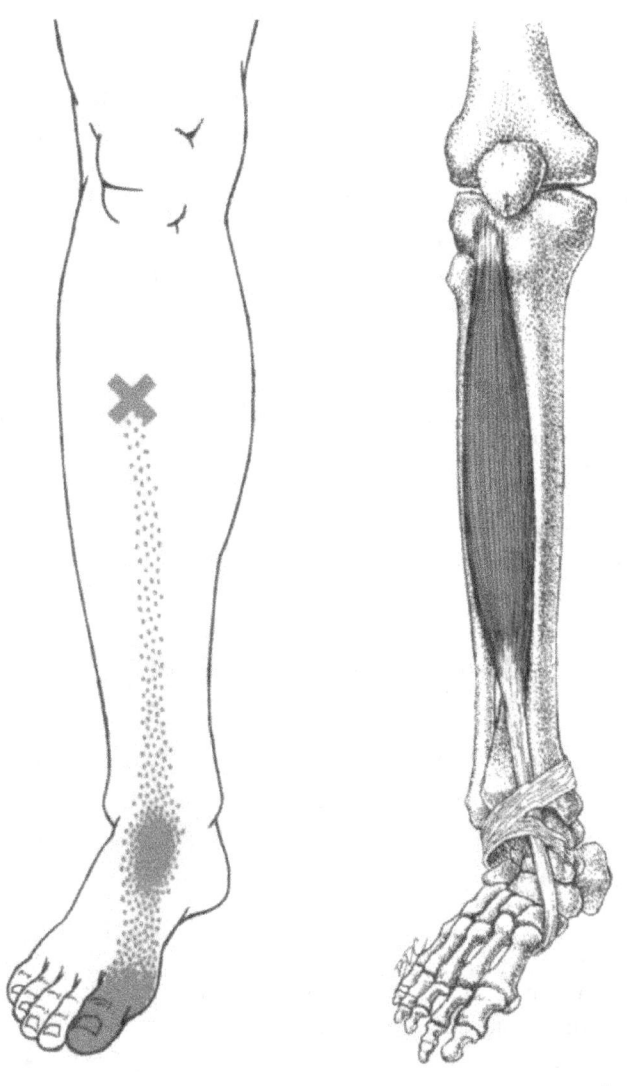

15 Biceps Femoris

Description:

This muscle lies at the back of the thigh and arises out of two heads. The muscle run down from the pelvis, towards the knee and form the hamstrings. The hamstrings are actually a mix of muscles and tendons. The actual muscle which pulls our leg back is the bicep femoris, which is the equivalent of the biceps in the arm, except in the legs everything is in reverse to the arm, with the biceps on the legs been on the back of the legs, whereas the biceps on the arms are in the front.

Function:

It helps to extend the leg backward. If you stand up and pull your foot up and back towards your bottom, then this is done via your ham bicep.

Symptoms:

Pain in the back of the thigh, knee, and calf.

Trigger Point Therapy:

It is located in the same place as acupuncture point urinary bladder 37 which is located six finger widths from the buttocks.

Simply feel around the back of the thigh and you should be easily able to locate this point. If confused, measure six of your finger widths and then take this measurement possibly via a measuring tape and drop it down from your lower buttock line to your mid-thigh.

The finger width measurements are based upon Traditional Chinese Medicine (TCM) "cun" measurement, whereby each finger width represents a "cun". In TCM the acupuncture points are worked out by measuring according to a person's individual "cun" measurement.

Chapter Five – Arms & Hands

16. Supinator

Description:
This muscle runs from the lower outer aspect of the upper arm down towards the front upper aspect of the lower arm.

Function:
This muscle rotates the lower arm outwards, in order to turn the palm inwards.

Symptoms:
Pain above the elbow and down the outer aspect of the forearm. It can also radiate pain down to the back of the hand above the index finger.

Trigger Point Therapy:
The trigger point is in the lower arm just under the inner elbow crease at the upper part of the inner aspect of the forearm, see diagram.

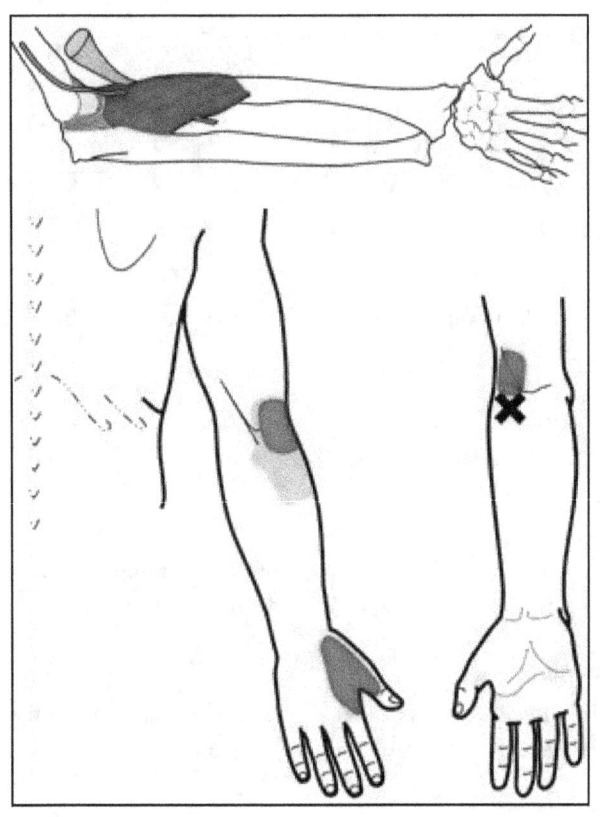

17. Extensor carpil radialis

Stomach trigger points

Description:

This arises from the outer aspect of the elbow and runs down to the base of the third and second fingers.

Function:

The extension and inwards bending of the wrist.

Symptoms:

Pain above the elbow joint and on the back of the hand. Sometimes involves stiffness and lack of mobility in the elbow.

Trigger Point Therapy:

This point is on the anterior aspect of the forearm several inches down from the elbow joint. So it's on the opposite side of the forearm to the supinator. So simply look at the upper front aspect of your forearm, coming from your elbow joint, and press around until you find a sensitive point.

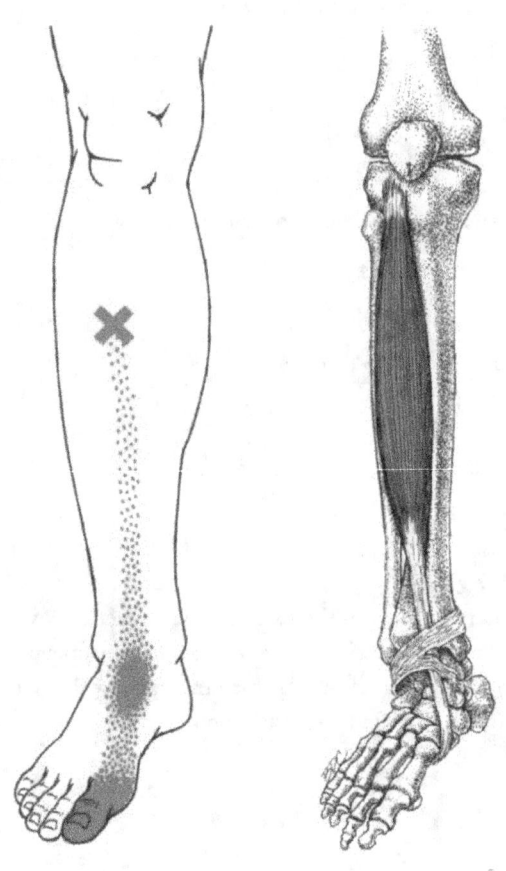

18. Middle finger extensor

Description:

This originates on the outer aspect of the elbow, moving downwards, via four tendons, into the base of the fingers.

Function:

It helps extend the fingers, in particular, the second and the third.

Symptoms:

Pain in the back of the hand and down the lower arm. This is often an aching pain and often there will be difficulty in moving the wrist and fingers.

Trigger Point Therapy:

This point is on the lateral aspect (side) of the forearm about two inches from the elbow joint. Simply have a feel around until feeling a sensitive point and then working in pressing and relieving the tension built up there.

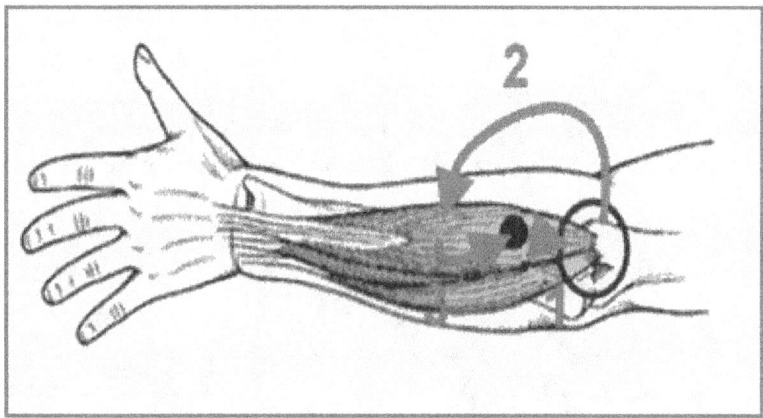

19. First interosseous

Description:

This muscle runs from the inner, upper surface of the bone at the base of the thumb and runs to the side of the index finger.

Function:

It helps to bend the index finger and pulls it over towards the thumb when the thumb is open.

Symptoms:

Pain and stiffness in the palm and on the back of the hand especially near the thumb and the index finger.

Trigger Point Therapy:

This point is really easy to find. Simply stretch out your thumb and your fingers so that your thumb is pulling away from your forefinger. What results is a triangular structure of flesh which lies between the forefinger and the thumb. Simply press around the midpoint of this fleshy triangle and you ill feel the point.

This is also a popular acupuncture/acupressure point and is known as Large Intestine 4 (LI 4) and it's also very good for working on expelling bacterial infections from the head. So if you start getting a head cold then pressurize this point for relief.

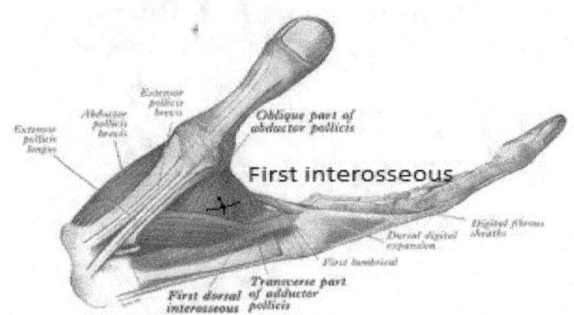

20. Abductor pollicis

Description:

This muscle runs from the base of the second and third carpal bones (the forefinger and middle finger) and it inserts into the inner side at the base of the thumb.

Function:

This draws the thumb and fingers together and is the main muscle to help the thumb bend.

Symptoms:

Pain and stiffness of the thumb especially in the outer aspect at the base of the thumb.

Trigger Point Therapy:

This trigger point is basically in the palm of the hand in the fleshy part near the thumb, just take a look at the diagram. If you feel around there you will easily feel a sensitive point. Simply press and release it with the thumb of your other hand.

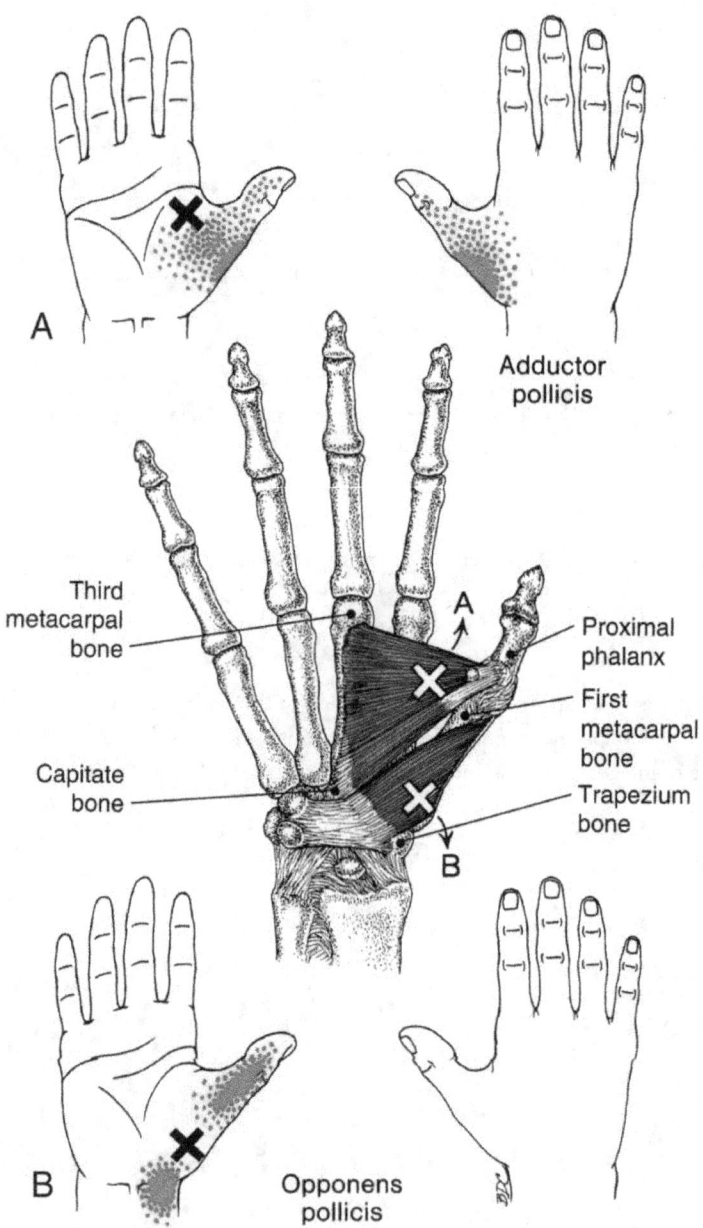

Notes

www.ingramcontent.com/pod-product-compliance
Lightning Source LLC
Chambersburg PA
CBHW030037230526
45472CB00002B/548